NATURE CURE FOR PAINFUL JOINTS

Natural measures for eliminating the pain and discomfort resulting from strains and minor injuries to joints (which often leads to rheumatism and arthritis), with simple tests for determining the amount of free-play movement within joints.

By the same author
HOW TO SAVE YOUR HEART
DIETS TO HELP KIDNEY DISORDERS

In this series
BANISHING BACKACHE AND
  DISC TROUBLES
HEADACHE AND MIGRAINE
  their causes and treatment
NATURE CURE FOR CONSTIPATION,
  APPENDICITIS, and other bowel disorders
NATURE CURE FOR PROSTATE TROUBLES
NATURE CURE FOR ARTHRITIS
SAVE YOUR TONSILS!
SELF-TREATMENT FOR HERNIA
SELF-TREATMENT FOR SKIN TROUBLES

Nature Cure for Painful Joints

Harry Clements N.D., D.O.

THORSONS PUBLISHERS LIMITED
Denington Estate, Wellingborough, Northamptonshire

First published July 1973

ISBN 0 7225 0231 1

Typeset by Specialised Offset Services Ltd., Liverpool and printed by Weatherby Woolnough Ltd., Wellingborough, Northants.

Contents

Foreword

Few people live out their lives without some disability to the joints of their body. It may be from some simple or serious strain or it may be the impact of violence of one kind or another. It may be from some kind of disease, particularly of arthritis, which seem to affect more and more people at the present time. Whatever the cause may be there is no doubt that joint complaints interfere with the physical efficiency of the individual and sometimes lead to secondary effects which are not always recognized and appreciated. The simple strained ankle, for example, if not properly restored to its normal condition can upset the posture of the whole body, and result in muscular tensions and a loss of nervous energy. It may upset the balance of the spine and be the unsuspected cause of backache.

One could go on giving examples of how joint complaints interfere with normal function in remote parts of the system, even to the point of affecting general health, but the main point to be emphasized is that the trouble in the joint or joints must be effectively removed and the full mobility of the joint restored. That this is not always done can easily be proven and the reader of this book may find that he is the possessor of a joint that is still limited in its use and in need of more restorative measures.

It is not an uncommon experience to find that many people, particularly as they grow older, accept a certain amount of limitation of movement in their joints — a perilous condition if they have rheumatism or arthritis in their system. Such a limitation usually stems from an accident or strain that has not been properly managed. It may well be that pain-killing drugs had eased the pain and that times had permitted the joint to fulfill most of the tasks assigned to it in the course of daily life, but with still a certain degree of immobility remaining. If the joint has not been put through its full movement during treatment, and very often this is the case, there is the risk that the infirmity will remain almost indefinitely. This is where the individual should play a more active part. He is able to test the full movement of the joint and he should not be satisfied until it has been restored. The writer has examined hundreds of cases and it is rare to find a person who has all the joints of the body working as normally as they should do.

While rheumatism and arthritis are now recognized as constitutional afflictions there is no doubt that strained and injured joints become the focal point for these diseases to develop. People who suffer from these complaints should make quite sure that every joint strain and injury is carefully managed and the joint returned to its normal condition. Unless the full movement of the joint is restored one may be sure that further troubles will develop.

It is true, of course, that the joints of the body are governed to a great extent by mechanical principles and that to fully appreciate their importance one must look at their assemblage from what one might call an engineer's point of view. This enables one to see how important mechanical adjustment is at all times so as to get the most efficient service out of them. But it would be wrong not to bear in mind that the joints of the body are an integral part of the whole system, depending on the circulation of the blood and other fluids, upon the nervous energy and the muscular power, and last but not least upon the nutriments that are brought to them, together with the eliminative processes which preserve the natural healthy balance.

The joints of the body are as dependent upon proper nutrition as any other part of the system, which is saying in effect that without adequate and proper food one cannot expect them to be healthy. Equally, one must see that the same thing applies to the treatment of strained and injured joints, and there is no doubt that when they are afflicted by rheumatism and arthritis attention to their nutrition is of the first importance. It is wrong to think that any kind of food that may be picked up at a supermarket will do: a wise selection must be made and the inclusion in the diet of the more whole and natural ones is indispensable.

In this book, which is meant for instruction rather than for mere reading, the repetition found is intentional, on the assumption that certain points need to be repeated rather than expecting the reader to refer back to previous paragraphs. The value which a reader will obtain depends on the information becoming a part of his thinking so that it can be applied when the occasion arises.

I.

What You Should Know About Joints

As we all know the bones of the skeleton are connected to adjacent ones and such connections are termed joints, or in the more strictly medical term, articulations. These joints are said to be immovable, slightly movable and freely movable. In the immovable ones such as we find in the skull the surfaces are separated only by a thin fibrous membrane, and so far as we are concerned in this discussion we shall pay little further attention to them. Where we find slight movement in joints such as in the spinal joints and the interpubic one the surfaces are united by tough and elastic fibrocartilages, all designed to give great strength. In the freely movable joints the surfaces are completely separated and the bones are covered with cartilage and held together with strong bands of fibrous tissue, known as ligaments. A very important structure of the freely movable joint is the synovial membrane which is the lubricating mechanism by which the various parts of the joint are lubricated.

The freely movable joints are the ones with which we shall be mostly concerned in dealing with joint complaints, and in these many soft tissues such as cartilage, fibro-cartilage, ligaments and synovial membrane, in addition to bone, enters into the structure. In addition we have the muscles which control the joint movements. These soft tissues are of particular interest to us in thinking about joint complaints since they, rather than the bones, sustain the effects of strains and injuries, and are the seat also of the changes which disease processes may bring about.

Let us, therefore, look a little more closely at these joint tissues so that we may understand the changes that may occur in them in the various complaints. Cartilage is a non-vascular structure. That is to say, it has no blood circulation through it and because of this it has to renew itself in other ways. It derives its nutrients partly from the bones to which it is attached and partly from the vessels of nearby synovial membrane. The elasticity of the cartilage enables it to act as a shock absorber to the forces of concussion through the joint and also at the same time plays an important part in the free movement of the joint. It apparently goes through a constant breaking down and building up process and is not therefore a stationary material set in the joints for the life-period.

The ligaments of the joint are peculiar to the movable joints. They serve the important purpose of holding together the surfaces of the bones and in the freely movable joints they form surrounding capsules. They are pliant and flexible, thus allowing freedom of movement while at the same time they are tough, strong and inextensible so as to stand up to very great strain. In spite of this they can be damaged by great violence and the healing process with ligaments is usually rather a slow one. Some ligaments are more elastic than others, depending on the nature of the function of the joints.

The synovial membrane of the joints is a thin, delicate connective tissue which secretes a thick liquid like the white of an egg and which is known as synovia. The synovial membrane differs in its structure in the various joints but it and its secretion play a vital part in the lubrication and movements of the joints. The synovial membranes are liable to be affected by the various forms of inflammation and the term synovitis is applied to such conditions.

These elementary facts about the structure of joints should be kept in mind when strains and accidents occur to them since it enables one to apply the necessary and proper treatment and to understand the effects which it may have upon the structures involved. It will also help one to understand how useless it may be to adopt methods of treatment which cannot possibly help in the healing process.

JOINT MOVEMENT

The efficiency of the body — and this is true of practically every physical activity that is undertaken — depends upon the unimpeded movement of the joints. The body is to a great extent a mechanical instrument with the normal movement of the joints as essential to its integrity. Every person knows — and may have experienced it in his own person — that the loss of normal function in any important joint will lead to the disturbance of the balance of the whole body and sometimes lead to great discomfort and disability. The health and efficiency of the whole musculo-skeletal system is more dependent upon the efficiency of the numerous joints than many people imagine; indeed, as osteopathy has shown, when the spinal joints are strained and limited in their movement even the general health of the individual may be affected.

The body joints are capable of many varied and complicated movements. Actually there are basically four kinds: gliding and angular, circumduction and rotation, but it is interesting to note that these movements may all be combined together so that an infinite number may be possible in one joint. One kind of motion only in a joint is not usually found. All movable joints have a certain amount of gliding movement; in some it is the only one. The angular movement occurs between the long bones giving one flexion and extension. In circumduction, which occurs in the hip and shoulder joints, the movement takes place between the head of the bone and the articular cavity, while rotation is a form of movement in which a bone moves round a central axis without undergoing any lateral displacement, as for instance in the rotary movement at the elbow joint.

While all these movements are of interest to the anatomist they are only of importance to the individual in that he can perform them properly. It is when these movements are limited and perhaps associated with stiffness and pain that his attention is drawn to them. This is a point of real importance that must always be remembered, particularly following the treatment of an accident or a strain: the full movement must be restored before one should be satisfied that the cure has been complete.

FREE-PLAY MOVEMENT
There is another very important feature about the joints which is often overlooked, even by some people who have to treat them in a professional manner, and that is what might be termed the free movement of them. This is a very difficult thing to describe because what the ordinary person regards as freedom within a joint is the movement that takes place when the joint is moved by the muscles. But about all normal joints there is a certain amount of loose movement when they are in a relaxed state. One can test this for oneself on the finger joints. When the joint is quite normal it can be made to move a little from side to side and to give one a general sense of looseness. If the finger joint has been strained or damaged or swollen this free-play of the joint will be lost and there may be stiffness

and pain. Yet in spite of this it may be possible to bend and straighten in what seems to be normal movement.

Practically every movable joint is possessed of this free-play when it is in a normal condition. And unless this free-play is restored to a joint after an injury of any kind a great deal of trouble will ensue. It is interesting to note that it has been the non-recognition of this fact that has led to the success of the old bone-setters in their treatment of joint troubles after the orthodox treatment had failed. When a joint is fractured or dislocated it is of course treated by the orthopaedic surgeon, to be followed usually by treatment by the physiotherapist. It has happened in many cases that after such treatment the free-play of the joint has not been restored, leaving a residue of stiffness and pain. The simple manipulation of the joint to restore the free-play will clear up both the stiffness and the pain and thus give to the manipulator probably an unfair amount of credit for his skill.

The same thing may happen after lesser injuries. The joints as we all know, are subject to sprains and strains and other forms of accidents and these of course do not need such skilled treatment: they may be treated by the individual himself after he has made a visit to the doctor for a diagnosis. He may do no more than just take pain-killing drugs and then get back to normal activity when the pain and stiffness has cleared up. These are the cases where the chronic aches and pains of the joints may be experienced, and practically all of them are due to the fact that free-play movement has not been restored.

It may well be that some exercises may be done to try to strengthen the muscles around the joint and in some cases these may have just the opposite effect for which they have been planned. The free-play movement of the joint is lost when the muscles are contracted, and in many cases of strains one of the real problems is to reduce the contraction. Sometimes, also, the muscles around an injured joint will go on guard, that is to say that the muscles will tighten to prevent movement in the acute stage. Again, this condition must be overcome before the normality of the joint can be restored.

It follows that in order to obtain free-play in the joint the muscles attached to the surrounding parts must be relaxed. Those who do manipulative work know that the relaxing of the muscles is the most important part of the technique since practically no force is then required to make the necessary adjustment; on the other hand conscious contraction of the muscles by the patient can completely defy all his skill.

The ordinary person can learn a valuable lesson from this fact and that is that relaxation of the muscles in connection with the movement of joints is just as important as muscular movements. The free-play movement in the joint can only take place when the associated structures are relaxed and as there is in all the joints of the body a certain degree of self-adjustment it can only operate when the parts are relaxed. Even when exercises are being used to tone up the muscles one should never forget that in order to get the most out of them a period of relaxation after the exercises must always be observed.

JOINT MUSCLES

The joints are stabilized by ligaments and to a certain extent by muscles. Well developed muscles give a good deal of protection to the joints and therefore undergo strain and even injury with less damage. The muscles also provide the power for the movement of the joints and the strength of the latter depend upon the former — a fact which must be obvious to everyone. The well-muscled individual is far less likely to suffer a strain in a particular joint than an individual whose muscles are flabby.

On the other hand individuals with very strong muscles may sometimes find them a hindrance when a strain has produced real damage since the contraction which takes place at such a time may be much more difficult to overcome when trying to establish the free-play of the joint essential to its normal state. For this reason athletes who do suffer such injury may be surprised that a less strong person may make a quicker recovery. In such cases measures must be taken to make sure that the powerful muscles are effectively relaxed otherwise the joint will remain impaired in function.

While it is true that the efficiency of the joints depend on the muscles it must also be remembered that if the joint is not working properly the muscles will lose their efficiency. In such a case the tone will go out of them and it will be found that ordinary exercise will not restore it. This can happen after any maladjustment of a joint which has deprived it of its free-play and massage and exercise will only cause disappointment until the trouble with the joint has been rectified. In any case of weakened muscles around a joint the place to look for the cause is in the joint itself. It has been well said that if we take care of the joints the muscles will take care of themselves.

JOINTS AND WEIGHT-BEARING

Apart from providing the human body with the power of locomotion, the joints play a very important part in weight-bearing and this, of course, complicates their function. Not all the joints of the body are involved in weight-bearing but several important ones are directly concerned, particularly those which bear relationship to the erect position. The ankles, the knees, the hips, the spinal joints are certainly of vital importance in this respect. And it does not take very much imagination to realise how much such weight-bearing adds to the stresses and strains which the joints must undergo in the course of daily living.

This brings us, of course, to the subject of body mechanics in which the joints play such an important part. The body has been likened to a machine in that it has to perform certain mechanical movements brought about by the action of muscles and joints, but the body does not resemble a machine in that it has the power of self-repair and self-adjustment. The body is, of course, in a constant state of self-adjustment with the joints responding to many forces including that of gravity. And in some ways the erect position of the body imposes a perpetual strain on the muscles and joints. Standing still is not without its strain upon the muscles and joints. The three bulks of weight, the head, the chest and the pelvis have to be held in balance and this is more difficult when the body is not in motion. That is why we find it easier to walk since in that motion there is a constant loss and gain in balance which is far less fatiguing.

When the body is well balanced in the erect position there is very little strain on the individual. All the weight-bearing joints are in alignment with the minimum of strain. But we see a very different picture when there is indifferent or bad posture. One or many of the joints may come under strain. We can easily visualize how the stooping posture may throw strain on the various joints of the spine and this in turn may affect the joints of the lower limbs. Of course, this also works in reverse; the damaged ankle or knee may cause the whole posture of the body to be upset and place under strain muscles and ligaments in remote parts of the system. In any case, where the bony surfaces of a joint are out of alignment the tendency will be for the cartilages of the joint to be under strain and in time to show signs of wear and tear. It is not age that causes wear and tear in joints but the effects of bad body mechanics on them.

Any joint which shows signs of wear and tear calls for attention to the posture of the whole body and the relationship to that joint of weight-bearing. This is particularly true in the case of arthritis where the joints are always at risk from faulty body mechanics and weight-bearing. This may often be shown, even in the early stages, by pain and swelling around the joint and the usual method of treatment is aspirin or one of the other pain-killing drugs. But alleviating the pain in this way without removing the strain will lead on to an incurable condition – a state so many arthritic patients find themselves in. It is true, of course, that arthritis is a constitutional disease, and that treating the joints only will not influence the course of the trouble but it is equally true to say that if a joint can be saved by effective treatment the lot of the sufferer, especially as far as locomotion is concerned, will be greatly relieved.

We must at all times so far as strains, injuries and complaints are concerned, bear in mind the effect of weight-bearing upon them and do everything possible to improve the posture of the whole body and body mechanics generally.

JOINTS AND SELF-ADJUSTMENT

It has been explained that in the normal joint there is always a certain amount of free-play and that the restoration of such a condition is a pre-requisite of full recovery. On the other hand it does sometimes happen that this free movement may prove to be an embarrassment. Most of us at one time or another have experienced a sudden catch in the joint that causes pain and immobility. It usually happens when one is in a relaxed position such as sitting down, and when quickly rising a catch takes place in the knee joint. Usually by wriggling the leg in an instinctive manner the catch is released and both the pain and immobility disappears. It may happen in other joints, the elbow, the shoulder and so on. It may also happen in the spine and in this case it may be more difficult to get it released. If it is not able to release itself the muscles around the joint may go into spasm and the individual may need help to get relief. When it happens in the spine it may lead to the popular belief that a disc has slipped. If the body is not able to make its own adjustment the large muscles of the spine may go into contraction and give rise to pain and great difficulty in straightening up the back. Relief will come with applied heat and the relaxation of the muscles when the joint will be able to move again freely.

A better understanding of the joints of the body and

their functions should help the ordinary person to make more effective use of his body in the course of daily living. Disabilities arising from joint complaints can be a real factor in undermining the health and fitness of the whole body, and may often be the basic cause of headaches, backache, and other unexplained pains, to say nothing of muscular and nervous disorders. Every effort should be made to maintain the integrity of the joints and to regain it in its fullest measure when it has been lost.

2.

How to Treat Injured Joints

In many ways we are more concerned about the proper management of simple injuries to joints rather than to the more serious ones, for the obvious reason that the patient is more likely to get professional advice and to take more care in the latter case. In addition, of course, the more serious case will be given enough rest to get relaxation of the involved muscles and the vital energy for the healing process. This is true of the weight-bearing joints, such as the knee and the ankle, where the proper initial treatment is likely to make all the difference in the restoration of normal function.

WATER TREATMENT

Nothing that has developed in science will give more help and relief in joint strains than the use of water for the purpose of applying heat and cold and thus affecting the circulation, the absorption of waste products and affording relaxation and the relief of pain. If such a strain has been serious enough to cause severe pain there is nothing that will give more relief than a full hot bath. The patient should stay in it until the pain has subsided and the muscles about the strained joint have been relaxed. This plan is far better than the taking of pain-killing drugs which may have side effects and complicate the issue by adding chemical agents to the blood circulation through the joints. The use of the cold compress should follow the hot bath.

The cold or cooling compress has been used in the treatment of many forms of illness and its uses date back to the time of Hippocrates, who advocated it, together with the free drinking of cold water. It has been superseded, unfortunately, by the use of the pain-killer drugs, which, although easier to handle certainly do not offer such effective and safe relief. Many people in using this simple compress measure do not realize that such an application can have profound physiological effects, but the fact is that it does do so. When the cold compress is applied to the skin, it causes contraction of the surface vessels, but it also causes dilatation of the deeper-lying ones and in this way we are able to influence the circulation. The cold compress has an important effect upon the nerve centres, setting forth nervous impulses which affect the local tissues, thus stimulating secretion, excretion, heat production and so on.

The cold compress can be used for the relief of pain and for stimulation in almost any part of the body but here, of course, we are mainly interested in its use in the case of joint complaints. The joint compress is in itself a very simple contrivance. It consists of a bandage wrung out in tap water and applied to the joint; in the case of the joints of the limbs the bandage may be wound around them. The bandage should be well covered with a heavy towel or similar material. Where there is a good deal of heat in the joint the bandage should be on the wet side and frequently changed. This is particularly true of the early stages of a strain when one is anxious to reduce the pain and the swelling. In the more chronic cases, where there is mainly stiffness and aching, the bandage should be wrung out fairly dry and then worn during the night. Incidentally, this is a very good way of inducing sleep which may be disturbed by a nagging joint.

When it is not possible or convenient to use the full hot bath the affected joint may be immersed for a short time in hot water before the cold compress is applied. In the case of the ankle, or the elbow, this is quite easy, but with other joints such as the shoulder a hot application may be applied before the compress. In the more chronic joint complaints where the trouble has gone on for some time this application before using the cold compress is very important. This may be very useful in treating the effects of strain of the knee joint and the hot water bottle can be used to maintain the heat for a longer period. Fill the hot water bottle half-full of hot water and then place it over the hot application which has been wound around the knee. Then cover with a thick towel to keep in the heat. Remove the application when it has cooled and quickly apply the cold compress.

In the treatment of arthritic joints the use of hot and cold water applications is essential, no matter what other form of treatment is being pursued. Where more than one joint is involved the hot bath should be employed and it can be made more effective in this case by adding to the water a pound of Epsom Salts, the kind that is used for bathing purposes. As in the treatment of ordinary injury to the joint, a cold compress may be applied to the affected part after the bath. At other times when using the hot and cold applications, use the hot application first, and maintain the heat for about ten minutes, then follow with the cold one. In arthritic joints there is usually a low grade of inflammation and it will be found that the cold compress will fairly quickly dry out. If it is applied just before retiring it can be left on for the whole of the night with beneficial results.

JOINT EXERCISE
Movement is, of course, the main function of joints. In a healthy joint such movement must be completely free.

When we say it must be free we mean that it must be much more than the ability to bend or rotate. The joint itself when it is relaxed must be loose and have no feeling of tension or tightness about it. One can demonstrate this for oneself by testing the middle joint of a normal finger. If the finger is totally relaxed it will be found that there is a certain looseness in the joint and that it can be moved in various directions and particularly sideways. This is what we mean by the free-play of a joint. If, on the other hand the finger is forcibly straightened out there will be no movement at all in the joint, and the same will be found when the joint has been injured or maybe swollen. This free-play movement exists only when the joint is relaxed and is the hall-mark of a movable joint.

In the ordinary way exercise is performed with the idea of affecting and strengthening the muscles and not so much attention is paid to the condition of the joint that may be involved. When a joint has been injured the muscles which surround it may be either swollen or go into spasm and as recovery takes place the muscles return more or less to normal. Exercise may then be undertaken to try to restore their muscular tone but if the free-play in the joint has not been restored the results of the exercise will not be satisfactory. For that reason one may find many cases where the injured joint and the muscles attached to it may never recover completely from the damage.

The reason for this is due to the fact that the tissues about the joint have never been completely relaxed and in consequence the body has not been able to make its normal adjustment. In some ways the more the muscles are exercised, when the free-play of the joint has not been properly restored, the less likely it is that this adjustment will be made. As we have already explained the normal joint is a loose one in which there is a movement that is not governed by the action of muscles. This movement can only be elicited when the joint is relaxed and from this view-point, paradoxical as it may sound, the chief purpose of joint exercise is to produce relaxation. Most joints of the body have a greater range of motion when the muscles attached to them are relaxed. This can be demonstrated in the wrist. If one tenses the muscles by clenching the fist the movement is considerably limited; if, on the other hand, all the muscles are relaxed then there is a very free movement in almost all directions.

KNEE JOINT TEST

The same applies to the knee joint. If the leg is pressed back and the muscles attached to the knee contracted the knee joint is firmly fixed. If, however, the knee is slightly bent it will be found that the muscles will be relaxed and that there will be a certain amount of free play in the knee joint. The same free movement in the knee joint can be elicited also in this way: sit on a chair and raise the leg so that the fingers of both hands can be laced around the knee. Allow the muscles of the lower leg to relax and then gently move the foot, with the ankle and the knee moving as freely as possible. The free-play of the knee joint can be plainly felt under the hands, but if the joint is not normal or under the effects of strain it will be found to be absent.

HIP JOINT TEST

The normal free-play of the hip joint can be demonstrated in a very simple way. Stand with the feet a few inches apart. Place the thumb and fingers over the hip joint, which can be plainly felt at the side and front of the upper thigh. Now raise the foot off the floor and allow the muscles to relax as much as possible. Then gently swing the foot in a circle and from side to side. If the joint is quite normal the free movement will be felt under the thumb and fingers. Unfortunately a great many people lose a percentage of the movement of the hip joint before they become aware of it, and when it has been lost it is not easy to regain. The hip joint is the great weight-bearing joint of the body and any loss in its function will be felt in the posture of the whole body.

SHOULDER JOINT TEST

The shoulder joint is often involved in strains and in view of the fact that many muscles play a part in the function of this joint it can be attended with prolonged discomfort and disability. The loss of the free-play in this joint often leads on to the 'frozen shoulder' trouble which may be difficult to eradicate unless it is taken in time. The test for free-play in this joint can easily be done by the ordinary person. Adopt the standing position, leaning slightly forward. Place the left hand on the right shoulder and allow the right arm to hang loosely. Shaking it a little will help in relaxing. Now swing the hand and arm in a small circle, at the same time feeling the free-play of the shoulder joint under the left hand. Only a small circle must be made; if the circle is enlarged the muscles of the shoulder will come into play and this will cancel out the loose movement. It is worth emphasizing that the muscles must be relaxed as completely as possible in order to elicit the free-play movement of any joint. This test will show whether treatment for the 'frozen shoulder' has been fully successful. Unless this free movement has been restored there will still remain a residue of the complaint that may lead on to trouble in the future.

ELBOW, WRIST AND HAND TEST

The elbow and the wrist may be tested and relaxed in a similar way. Grip the upper arm with the left hand and then gently rotate the wrist so that all the muscles of the forearm are relaxed. Those who suffer from tennis elbow will not, of course, be able to relax these muscles, and, again, treatment for this complaint is not fully satisfactory until this free movement has been restored.

There are many joints in the hand that may be subject to strain or injuries. Few people seem to understand that in the well-developed hand there is an arch just as there is in the foot. When the hand is quite normal this arch may be tested by pressing the hand flat on a hard surface such as a table and then releasing the pressure. It will be seen that the hand rises to a small arch. This arching process may be lost when the hand has been injured or strained and one or more of the joints are not functioning properly. This may be accompanied by pain in the hand and it may well be the condition which precedes the deformity of the fingers through the deposits around the finger joints. Restoring the arching process of the hand by pressure and relaxation, as described above, is a good way, not only of testing the joints, but also of relieving the tension in the various muscles.

The foot, like the hand, is composed of many joints, and its arch, of course, is much more pronounced. But it operates in very much the same way. The normal foot tends to flatten under the weight of the body and to re-form its arch when the foot is taken off the ground. When it has been strained or injured it tends to lose this flexibility and when this has been lost the foot becomes deficient in its propulsion powers. This can occur after a strain affecting the ankle joint since some of the joints of the foot invariably share in the strain. This can have a very serious effect upon the locomotion of the whole body since in walking and running the propulsive power of the foot plays a very important part.

Foot complaints arising from strains and injuries are very common and in many cases the treatment has not been effective in restoring the free-play of the ankle and the other joints. The tense, aching foot is a concomitant of this condition and is as common as it is troublesome. We must remember also that the foot is encased in shoes which may limit in some way the freedom of the joints and play no small part in the aching feet syndrome with 'my-feet-are-killing-me' symptoms.

THE FOOT-BATH
One of the best ways of relaxing foot and ankle joints is by using the foot-bath. A receptacle is needed that is large enough to allow the foot to lie flat on the base of it. Fill the vessel with hot water and then put the weight on the

foot to flatten the arch and then release it to allow the arch to re-form. The effect of the hot water on the foot tissues helps in the relaxation process and at the same time will help the body in its normal adjustment of the various joints. Those who suffer from tense, aching feet will find this treatment very helpful in relieving the troublesome symptoms.

BACKACHE

Some of the most important joints in the body are found in the spine and the same principle of the free-play movement applies to them. They are, of course, much more limited in this way than many of the joints of the limbs, but still such movement is important and gives rise to various symptoms when it is lost. When the spine is in normal condition it is very flexible and this means that the extensive system of muscles which are attached to it are responsive to every movement of the body. Today very few occupations enable the individual to use the spine to its proper extent, and, in consequence, this flexibility may be considerably reduced. As a result the spine becomes stiff and many of the spinal muscles lose their tone. This means that the free-play movement of the spine will be lost and aches and pains will be felt in the back region. As many people know — perhaps from personal experience — backache has become the universal complaint of the industrial society. At any time in this country it is estimated that a million people suffer from this trouble, which may be severe enough to interfere with their work, and this of course, leaves out of account the many more who suffer in this way but not be severe enough to warrant medical attention or absence from work.

The loss of the flexibility of the spine and free-play of its joints places the spine in a precarious condition. An unusual or sudden movement of the body produces what is known as a 'crick in the back' and from then onwards the backache becomes a real problem. What has really happened is not always clear. The 'slipped disc' idea became a convenient rather than a correct one, and while in a few cases the discs were involved, in the majority of them it may not be the right explanation. It is more likely to be due to a loss of flexibility of the whole spine with the loss of the free-play of the joints, together with the loss of resiliency of the muscles and other spinal structure. The condition tends to correct itself with rest and relaxation, but as this may not make any fundamental change in the condition of the spine the same thing can happen again at almost any time.

Loss of flexibility in the spinal structures must in the long run lead to changes in the discs. The discs are shock absorbers, and they are under compression from the muscles. The health of the discs depends upon movement for the preservation of their elasticity, which, of course, the stiff spine denies to them. Add to this the force of gravity on the whole spinal column and we see how the discs must in time lose their elasticity and become hardened and thinned. It is this thinning process that finally gives rise to the disc lesions. Then we are in a vicious circle. The loss of flexibility of the spine has undermined the resiliency of the discs and with the changes in the discs the restoration of the spinal flexibility may be very difficult if not impossible.

TREATMENT OF SPINAL JOINTS

In order to maintain free-play of spinal joints the spine must be treated as a whole. It must be regarded as a flexible instrument with many components entering into its total relationship. It is rarely a question of one joint in the spine being the sole repository of the trouble: the integrity of the whole maintains the integrity of the part. In the management of joint complaints in the spine we must restore the full free movements of all of them and as with the other joints of the body, relaxation is the important point to consider. It is true that rest is usually prescribed for such complaints but much more conscious effort must be made to induce it than is usually the case.

First of all the muscular tension must be relieved and for this purpose nothing is more effective than the use of the hot bath. It should be taken quite hot and the sufferer should stay in it until it cools down. In some cases it may be prolonged by adding hot water if the pain is severe. The hot bath is an effective way of relieving pain and is very much better than the taking of the various pain-killing drugs. It may be indulged in a couple of times a day if necessary.

A great deal may be done by the individual himself in the freeing of the spinal joints and relieving the muscular tensions of the back. It is worth noting that many people live a good deal of their lives without really straightening their backs. In many occupations and in various everyday pursuits the body is in the position of flexion, that is, in the slightly bending forward position. This applies to the majority of workers in an industrial society, and such a position puts a strain on the back muscles in particular. The same is true of many hobbies such as gardening, and driving a car. When such a person is tired at the end of the day he returns home to recline in an easy chair, which accentuates the position his body has been in for most of the day. By then his body is fixed in the flexion position and possibly tense from strain. The night's sleep spent in a soft, yielding bed does little to relieve the tense, strained muscles, especially, of course, in middle and later life when the habit has been firmly implanted and the body less resilient. In the course of time, and if nothing is done to remedy the condition, certain parts of the spine will become stiff and the discs will harden and shrink in size.

CORRECTIVE EXERCISE

This condition can be prevented and corrected if taken in time. What must be done is to re-establish the proper relationship between the extensor and flexor muscles of the back. The simplest corrective exercise to accomplish this is to lie flat on the back on the floor. It must be on an unyielding surface so that relaxation of all the muscles can take place. It may sound an easy thing to do but many people who have by daily habits fixed their spines in the forward position will find it quite difficult. This is the optimum position for the relaxation of the back muscles and after a few minutes one is aware of the fact that the muscles are 'letting go'. Those who do have pain and tension at one particular part of the spine may feel that it has increased when first assuming the position, but this will gradually be relieved. It will help matters if the individual will concentrate his mind on the idea that the muscles must relax.

Changing the spine from the vertical to the horizontal position takes the strain off the large muscles or guy ropes, and this will allow the body to make its own adjustment. Those who practise manipulative therapy know that this self-adjustment is constantly taking place and that the main part of their work is to relax the muscles so that this adjustment may take place. It is true that there is always the exceptional case which may need help in such an adjustment but the exception only proves the rule. So many cases of spinal joint complaints arise through very little applied violence; a slight turn of the body, a little strain in moving an object and suchlike happenings often prove the time for the trouble to appear which comes as unexpectedly as it is painful.

The main point to emphasize in endeavouring to restore the essential free-play of a joint is that relaxation is the important factor. It is not a question of trying to force movement in a joint by the application of some kind of muscular exercise; it is an attempt to relax the various structures so that the body can make its own adjustment. It needs mental as well as physical effort to relax and we must know what we are trying to achieve through its application. We know that in joint complaints we have to restore to joints their complete freedom of movement and it is surprising how much it helps a person if he has his objective clearly in mind.

JOINT MOVEMENT AND ARTHRITIS

Arthritis is perhaps the commonest of all afflictions in this country and it has been estimated that few people will escape it after reaching middle life. As one or more of the joints of the body are affected in this disease we can say that only a very small minority of people will escape some infirmity of the joints. It is true that with the developing skill of the surgeon artifical joints may now be possible, but even the greatest enthusiast for such a procedure would agree that to save one's own joints is a much better plan. And one can say from practical experience that a great deal can be done in this way if the strains and injuries to which the joints are subject are carefully managed in their early stages. The person suffering from arthritis should bear in mind that he must pay even more attention to early and careful treatment of joint complaints than someone with no arthritis in himself or in his family.

Unfortunately many people think that because arthritis cannot be cured, when a diagnosis of it is made something has happened that cannot be reversed. This has happened in many cases where careful treatment would have been of much help. It often happens when a person has a pain in a joint that an X-ray will be advised. The X-ray may show early signs of arthritis and the pain will be regarded as the result of the disease. The attitude then is that nothing more can be done. The patient may also be told that the trouble is linked to wear and tear which will confirm the hopelessness of the situation.

This defeatist attitude is more destructive of the patient's ability to help himself, or get help, than the disease itself. In so many of these cases the complaint, and particularly the pain, is due to some joint strain or injury that has not been properly treated and where the essential free-play of the joint has not been restored. It may well be that in many cases the pain may be wrongly attributed to arthritis, since there is some doubt that the disease causes so much pain. We would not go all the way with Dr Mennel, who in his book *Joint Pain*, says: 'There is, of course, no anatomical, physiological or pathological reason why osteoarthritis should give rise to pain. If there were, it would be reasonable to tell a patient that not too much can be done to alleviate the symptoms other than relieving the joint of weight bearing, if it is in the lower limbs, or from use, if it is in the upper limbs. Certainly, there is a wearing away of the hyaline cartilage in an osteoarthritic joint, and when it is gross, it may be that bone might rub upon bone and give rise to pain symptoms. But so long as the articulating bony surface is covered by cartilage at all, there is no reason why pain should arise from this simple wearing-away process, since, of course, the hyaline cartilage does not have any nerve supply.'

Whether this reasoning is completely right or not it is, of course, difficult to argue, but there is no doubt at all that many cases of osteoarthritic joints can be relieved of painful symptoms by the treatment advocated here for the treatment of strained or injured joints. In any case it can be said that nothing but good can result from the treatment of arthritic joints by means of hydrotherapeutic measures and the restoration of free-play in the joints. Until that has been done no one should be willing to accept this idea that osteoarthritis is the sole cause of the pain and discomfort.

POSTURE AND JOINT PAIN
The weight-bearing joints of the body like the ankle, knee and hip are directly involved with posture – the way in which people stand, walk, and generally move around, and strain and injuries of all kinds are liable to cause more trouble than in other joints. A vicious circle is set up in this way: bad posture invariably adversely affects the joints and joint disability disturbs the body equilibrium. The deranged knee will cause the person to limp and this will upset the balance of the rest of the body. On the other hand, faulty posture will affect the weight-bearing func-tioning of certain joints and this will make them suscep-tible to strain and in the long run possibly arthritis. We

have only to watch people in the streets and observe the carriage of their bodies to see how common bad posture is and what an important factor it must be in undermining the integrity of the various weight-bearing joints.

THREE EXERCISES

There are three exercises that may be done both for the purpose of testing the efficiency or otherwise of the posture of the body and of correcting disabilities that may exist.

1. Lie flat on the floor with feet pressed against the wall. It is important to notice that the back of the head contacts the floor and that to achieve this the chin is kept well tucked in. Reach above the head with both hands, keeping them in line with the body. Stretch the arms as much as possible and if this is done forcibly enough the buttocks and the lower spine will be lifted off the floor. Hold the position for a few minutes and then relax. Repeat a few times.

2. Stand in a doorway. Reach with the hands to the top of the door frame. Now, keeping hold on the frame, walk in very short steps as far forward as possible and then backwards. If this exercise is done properly it is one of the best ways of improving the posture; it pulls up the shoulders and ribs and stretches the abdominal muscles as well as the spine. It also stretches the finger joints and if one walks back far enough it stretches the toes and the arches of the feet.

3. Stand about a foot or fifteen inches from the wall. Reach with the hands as high as possible up the wall. Now allow the abdomen to fall towards the wall. This will bring the feet up on to the toes and the stretching movement will be felt in the lower back, which will be pulled forward. Still holding this position press the heels down on to the floor, stretching the calf muscles. Alternatively, press down one foot at a time giving a kind of sea-saw effect across the pelvis and the lower spine.

These exercises can be used both to test and improve

the posture. It will often be found that if there are one or more joints in the body that are not working efficiently their presence will be revealed. Stretching the way suggested will test the shoulders, the spine, the knees and the ankles, and if any of these joints have been strained or injured at some time the deficiency in the movement will be shown. At the same time these exercises, if practised for a while, will help to correct such disabilities. They will be of the greatest value to those who suffer from arthritis, especially if practised in the early stages of the complaint when every possible thing should be done to preserve the integrity of the joints. Of course, when the disease has advanced and some of the joints have been badly damaged, the full movements demanded by the exercises may be impossible. But, even so, an attempt should be made to do them within the capacity of the patient since they can be so helpful in preventing further deterioration.

NUTRITION AND JOINT COMPLAINTS

It has often been observed that wild animals and some domestic ones that have not entirely lost their natural instincts, not only rest their limbs when they are injured, but also refuse to take food of any kind. Certainly this is true of any kind of injury that has been severe enough to break a bone, or to tear the flesh, but even in minor ones, particularly if there has been any kind of shock, the same self-discipline is fairly rigidly applied. We do not, of course, know the reason for this, if indeed reason enters into the matter. The animal must be complying with some physiological response that has been called into action in order to deal with the emergency. We do not give animals credit for awareness in such conditions and we therefore assume that the response is purely of physical origin. Philosophically speaking, it makes sense because there would not have been survival if nature had not developed some kind of protective and curative function within the animal body to operate under such conditions since in the circumstances it would not have the intelligence to cope with such situations. It is sometimes overlooked that the best example of the existence of the *vis medicatrix naturae*, the healing power of nature, is to be found in the body of the animal where it operates with efficiency in the healing of disease and the repair of injuries which would otherwise threaten animal existence.

It is often wrongly assumed that these facts do not apply to the human body; that we have so radically changed our life and environment that they do not apply to man. The simple fact is that such a change has made very little difference and that we are equally dependent today on the inherent power of the body to take care of our illnesses and injuries as we were when we lived a more natural life. It is a mistake to think that medicines can ursurp this function of the body; what they do is to relieve pain and abate symptoms and in some measure change the pattern of the disease reaction. People often talk loosely and without much reason about the word 'cure', implying that we do possess such a thing and that in the future we shall find others for all our ills. But let them try to count on the fingers of their hands the number that they have in mind of any agents that will totally eliminate from our midst the various forms of disease. Even those who are the most enthusiastic advocates of medical progress have to admit that medicines are still only handmaidens of nature: that in the last analysis it is the body's power of healing that leads finally to recovery.

In all the great progress that has been made in surgery we still have to reckon with the necessary co-operation of nature in the final healing process. No matter what operation is performed from the least minor to the major ones such as organ transplants, unless the recuperative power of the body is able to be maintained the work of the surgeon will have been in vain. The same applies to accidents and injuries where the skill of the surgeon is life-saving, and yet it still remains true that unless the healing power of the body is able to function the efforts of the surgeon will have been in vain. The mending of the broken bone, the healing of a cut or open wound depends on the healing power of the body and the most that we can do is to see that nothing is done to hinder it.

IMPORTANCE OF NUTRITION

Modern knowledge of the function of joints teaches us that to best influence their welfare and help them in recovery from injury and ailments we should pay proper attention to their nutrition and this means attention to food and food habits. Some people may feel that strains and ailments of joints need little thought about diet and its relationship to their recovery but this is a mistaken idea. There is no doubt that as far as prevention is concerned nutrition plays a very important part. Weak joints are far more likely to be strained and to suffer from ailments of many kinds. And weak joints are often due to the fact that the body is not being properly nourished by good and suitable food. The various structures and tissues of the joints such as the muscles, ligaments, synovial membranes and so on, are only as strong as the whole body is strong and unless the blood supplying these joint structures bring to them the elements of nutrition by which their strength and resistance can be built up we cannot expect them to be strong and healthy. As confirmation of this fact we all know that in the gross deficiency diseases, such as rickets and scurvy, both due to errors of nutrition, the joints and the joint structures are badly affected.

In injuries and strains of joints we should remember that the whole system is involved in some way. Of course, if the strain is very slight very little notice may be taken of it but if it is sufficient to make the sufferer 'feel sick' as the expression goes, then attention should be paid to the question of diet. The body has received a shock sufficient enough to affect and upset the digestive organs and to load them with a heavy meal will be to court indigestion. The joint requires rest and so do the digestive organs. It will be found most helpful to take very little solid food for the following twenty-four hours; warm lemon juice and honey drinks and fruit juices is probably the best plan.

In many cases where sufferers complain that they are constantly straining one or other of the joints of the body, particularly the ankles, some thought should be given to the possibility that the nutrition of the whole body has not been suitably adjusted and it is more than likely that too much reliance has been placed on the refined and over-prepared foods. A diet made up largely of foods like white flour, white sugar, extracted fat and the articles that are made from them, with an insufficiency of the natural foods, the fruits and salads, will undermine the health and strength of the tissues of the joints and prevent them from standing up to the normal strains of everyday life. It is not such a far cry from weakened ankles to white flour and white sugar as many people may think.

'PURE, WHITE AND DEADLY'

Such a conclusion should not surprise people. These refined foods are being looked upon by the medical profession with far more questioning eyes as to the part which they play in the causation of many forms of disease. Animal fats and concentrated ones like butter and margarine are thought by some authorities to be a major factor in the causation of coronary attacks, and a professor of nutrition places the blame for these tragic attacks on the use of white sugar. He calls it 'pure, white and deadly' and offered a good deal of evidence to show that it could also be responsible for many other conditions of ill health. It has been shown by many authorities that the excessive use of the refined foods, particularly white sugar, plays a large part in the causation of gout, and this disease, as we all know, directly affects the joints. Nature Cure practitioners have often shown that the withdrawal of white sugar and other refined foods from the diets of people suffering with arthritis will relieve its pains and tend to prevent its further development.

If people want to have strong healthy bodies with joints and muscles able to stand up to strains and minor injuries, all these foods should be excluded from the diet, or, at least cut down to a minimum. This is especially true of white sugar, which is taken in such excessive quantities because of its appeal to the palate. The drinking of tea, coffee and soft drinks, all of which are overloaded with sugar, is the main source of the trouble. If we add to this the sugar taken in sweets and puddings we get some idea of the excessive amount that the ordinary person may consume. Sugar is, in fact, a stimulant, and after it has been used for some time it may easily become an addiction that is very hard to break. And because many people believe the fallacious notion that it is a source of energy they see no reason for limiting its use. But to continue using this pure, white and deadly article so recklessly is to court disaster with the general health and also with the joints of the body.

In order to keep the muscles and joints of the body in good condition and able to bear the strains imposed upon them the body must have a balanced diet in which all the elements of a complete diet are to be found, and it is just as important that the foods themselves are as nearly as possible in their natural state. One of the best ways of arranging a balanced diet which will include all the protein, carbohydrates, vitamins and mineral salts is to plan it along the following lines. One meal should consist mostly of raw ripe fruit. Breakfast time is a good time for it. To this add milk and wholewheat products as may be desired. For another meal, which may be the midday one, take mostly raw green salad comprising all kinds of raw vegetables. To this add nuts, wholewheat products, potatoes, rice, and suchlike starchy dishes. For the third meal, which may be taken in the evening take mostly cooked vegetables to which may be added lean meat, fish, eggs, cheese, or if a vegetarian, suitable substitutes.

The important thing in this plan is to make quite sure that the fruit, salads and cooked vegetables are given priority and not the other way round. So long as that order is preserved one may add all kinds of other foods to each meal but always remembering that simple plain ones are the best for building up good health. While it is true that the muscles and joints cannot be made strong without exercise it is also true to say that unless the nutrition is sound and well balanced, exercise will be of little avail.

3.
The Chief Joints Involved in Injuries

JOINTS OF THE SPINE

Millions of people suffer from various forms of backache and in most cases this means that the joints of the spine are suffering from the effects of strains or minor injuries. People used to speak of the spine as if it were one massive bone, but, in fact, it is a series of bones which functioning together gives to the spine great flexibility. It is this flexibility that gives to the body its ability to adapt itself to all kinds of movements, and it is the loss of this flexibility that leads to all kinds of disabilities.

The flexibility of the spine is dependent upon the normal functioning of its joints and these are more numerous than many are aware. In addition to those in the spine itself there are those of the heads of the ribs where they articulate with the spine. Every time we breathe in and out movement takes place in these joints and when they may be injured or strained they can give rise to pain and discomfort that may easily be mistaken for more serious complaints. The flexible spine helps in the movement of these joints whereas a rigid spine limits them and, incidentally, limits the capacity of the chest and lungs.

FUNCTION OF THE DISCS

The most flexible parts of the spine are in the lower back or lumbar region and in the neck or cervical area. It is in these areas where strains and injuries take place and where the so-called slipped disc is found. So much attention has been focused on the discs that it is generally overlooked that this is essentially a joint complaint. We often speak of disc lesions, prolapsed disc and herniated disc, and this gives the false impression that only the disc is involved in the trouble. In fact, the disc is an elastic ring of cartilage fitted between the surfaces of two bones which allows for movement and gives overall flexibility to the spine. When, through injury, or some other cause, one of the discs becomes strained, the flexibility of the whole spine may be affected and this will mean that all the muscles of the back will not be able to function normally. This will tend to limit the movements of the body and if the trouble is not corrected the lower region of the spine takes on a certain amount of rigidity.

The discs of the spine also act as shock absorbers so that when they are involved in strains and injuries the effect may be felt throughout the system. The discs are very much involved in all the movements of the spine and their health and integrity depends upon such movements. When this movement becomes limited there is a tendency for rigidity to set in and the discs will suffer in consequence. If this condition continues into the chronic stage it may be said that the discs are degenerating.

The point is, of course, that the damage to the disc has put the joint out of its normal function. And this also will mean that, as with other joints in the body, the adjacent structures also will be affected. The ligaments may harden and shorten and the associated muscles will lose their tone and efficiency. A joint not functioning normally in the spine can throw the whole of it out of balance and indeed, upset the posture of the body. No other joints of the body can have a more disturbing effect upon the rest of the system than one or more of the spinal joints when they are not functioning normally.

If the sufferer has a tendency to rheumatism or arthritis, we may be sure that unless the joints have been restored to normal function the disease is most likely to settle there and full recovery will be greatly impeded. The arthritis will make movement in the spine much more difficult and this will directly affect the discs; they will lose their resiliency and become thinner and harden. If branches of the sciatic nerve become involved than sciatica may develop which will greatly add to the patient's suffering and disability.

NECK JOINT DISORDERS

These conditions which are often seen in the lumbar region of the spinal column may also be found in the joints of the neck. Here they cause great problems for the individual and considering the number of people seen around wearing cervical collars, the trouble must be on the increase. The upper part of the spine is particularly liable to shocks and strains; one has only to think of the jars and jolts of vehicle riding to see how much the neck must be affected under such conditions. Unfortunately, too, this part of the spine seems to be susceptible to the development of arthritis, which can be the cause of much physical distress.

Just as pains and injuries to the joints of the lower spine may set up pains in the legs, so too, the same thing may happen in the joints of the neck. The pains may radiate down the arms to the finger tips, sometimes causing tingling. The pains may also run up over the scalp and in some cases headaches may occur as a result.

When the joints of the upper spine are affected in this way the sufferer may be afflicted with inexplicable bouts of dizziness. In this respect we should remember that the regulation of the balance of the body is closely related to the movements of the neck in its efforts to maintain the position of the head over the centre of gravity. If there is a failure of response in this way a short spell of dizziness may occur. Free movement of the joints of the neck is essential to good posture and physical well-being.

The two joints or articulations at the top of the spine are very important and the significance of their free movement is often overlooked. They give us the free nodding movement of the head and the easy rotation of it, without involving the rest of the spine. Many complex ligaments and muscles, which are liable to strains of many kinds, are involved in these movements. The twenty-odd muscles associated with these joints are often seats of tension which may be of physical or mental origin, and such tensions may cause discomfort in other parts of the body.

There is no doubt that when we are considering the health and welfare of the body the spinal joints take on a special significance. When through strains and other injuries they lose their free movement the whole system is liable to suffer. For that reason such conditions should never be neglected. In some cases professional help may be needed to restore these joints to their normal functions but there is also no doubt that the individual can do a great deal to help himself in such circumstances. In the very early stages of spinal joint strains the use of hot baths and hot fomentations with proper rest and relaxation will often allow the body to make its own adjustment and thus overcome the trouble. As the muscles surrounding the affected joint or joints will be under strain, gentle movements may be required to restore their normal tone and resistance. But above all, it must be seen that the flexibility of the whole spine has been restored and that each joint has regained its natural free movement.

THE SHOULDER JOINT

There are very few people who have not suffered the discomfort and inconvenience of a strained or injured shoulder joint. The number of ways in which the shoulder joint may become strained or injured are almost legion and many of them come rapidly to mind. Even the carrying of heavy shopping bags can be a cause of strain; the pulling of a heavy dog on a leash may be another. Throwing an object may strain the joint and even shifting the gear lever on a car may do the same. Almost every individual who

have suffered in this way will have his own pet theory of
how it happened. Whatever the cause may have been, there
is no doubt that it is a very painful affliction that greatly
limits the capacity of the arm that is involved.

Many different diagnoses may be used in the case of the
painful shoulder. The terms bursitis, neuritis, neuralgia,
fibrositis, are often used to describe the condition and of
more recent date the term 'frozen shoulder' is used.
Whatever we call it, it certainly is a very painful affliction
that can give the patient a lot of trouble. Generally
speaking it follows a strain or some minor injury which has
been minor enough to have been largely forgotten.

Let us briefly consider the shoulder joint. The shoulder
itself is a bony, yoke-like arrangement, hung across the top
of the chest. It is not directly attached to the spine. This
girdle serves as a support for the arms which are fitted into
it by ball-and-socket joints. And, of course, it provides
attachments for the many muscles which move the arms
through the various planes. This arrangement enables the
arms to move freely and purposefully in a wide range
without bringing any undue pressure on the upper part of
the chest, where the heart and lungs are situated.

The collar bones extend from the shoulder blades to the
sternum, the bone in the front of the chest, and they form
the only connection between the shoulder and the arms
and trunk. Their function is to give support for the
shoulder joints, and act also to keep the shoulders free
from the chest. The arms, like the thighs, are fitted into
ball-and-socket joints with loose capsule ligaments, to
allow free motion of the arms.

It is easy to understand how an injured or restricted
shoulder joint affects a great many muscles of the body.
Numerous muscles are involved in just the free hanging
position of the arms, but when it comes to the great
number of movements that can be made with the arms,
with the shoulder joint as the pivotal point, this number
has to be greatly increased. When the shoulder joint is
working normally few people realize how many muscles

they are using when the arms are going through their usual movements in lifting, and doing all the various movements that are expected of them. It is when something goes wrong that it brings home to the patient the importance of the shoulder joint in all the daily activities. Pain and discomfort may be felt in the muscles of the back and shoulders, and it may even spread up into the neck. All the movements which we take for granted in the normal way will become difficult. Reaching with the hand behind the back, brushing hair, cleaning teeth, and even shaving, will be attended with difficulty and discomfort.

One of the most troublesome of the symptoms of the injured or strained shoulder joint is the discomfort which it causes when the patient is lying down, which of course deprives him of essential rest and sleep. In some cases the discomfort may not be felt so much during the day but returns at night time, and in most cases sleeping with the arm and shoulder resting on the bed gives rise to a great deal of pain.

It is well to remember that because there is such a wide range of movement in the shoulder joint it is possible to carry on most of the day's activities while there is still a good deal of limitation in such movements. Generally speaking, the patient lives in hope that it will get better of its own accord and is inclined to wait patiently for this to happen. In time, the lack of free movement becomes less noticeable and by a little compensation on other parts of the body the partly frozen shoulder may not seem to be too much of an impediment. But there is a real danger in such a situation. If there should be some tendency in the patient, or maybe in his family, to rheumatism or arthritis, then this restricted shoulder joint is very likely to become the focal point for the complaint. And if osteoarthritis does settle in the shoulder joint it can become a very real disablement. Every thing possible should be done to prevent it, and there is no doubt that if the joint is fully restored to its normal free movement after injury or strain a real step in prevention will have been made.

There is a very good way of testing the freedom of the shoulder joint and at the same time helping in its restoration. To treat the right shoulder joint: stand by a chair and place the left hand on the back of it for support. Then bend the body forward, allowing the right hand to hang as freely as possible. It will be noticed that in all cases of strains and injuries the tensed muscles will make this rather difficult and one must try to consciously relax them. Using a weight in the hand – the family iron is an admirable one – will be found to be useful. To do this part of the exercise properly is very important. One must persist until the arm is relaxed and hanging without any muscular effort.

When this condition has been achieved a swinging movement is done with the iron but at the same time the relaxed state of the muscles must be maintained. Allow the weight to swing backwards and forward several times and then allow it to swing in a circle, first one way and then the other. After this has been done several times, allow the arm to rest and then rotate the wrist using as little muscular effort as possible. This will rotate the bone of the upper arm in its socket.

During the whole of the exercise the mind must be kept on the shoulder joint, sensing, as it were, its free movement. This exercise will be found to be very useful in connection with the use of the hot baths and hot applications which are essential to the treatment of shoulder complaints. Such disorders are now becoming almost as frequent as the so-called slipped disc and in some cases as difficult, or even more difficult, to manage. Persistent efforts are often needed to overcome them.

THE KNEE JOINT
The knee joint is often involved in strains and other minor injuries, the treatment of which formed some of the contention between Sir Herbert Barker and the medical profession. A good deal of publicity is often given to knee injuries in which the cartilages are damaged, since they

generally arise through sporting events, such as football, in which the knee joint seems to be particularly vulnerable. The synovial membrane of the knee joint is sometimes damaged or affected by rheumatism, leading to what is known as synovitis, and when the bursa of the knee joint is injured, perhaps by too much kneeling, the term 'housemaid's knee' may be applied to it.

The knee is the largest joint in the body, but in spite of its size it has certain mechanical disadvantages. It is, of course, directly involved in the weight bearing of the body and so long as the knee is held in the vertical position it is immensely powerful and able to undergo great strain. But it is not so well equipped to meet the stress of rotation and sidewise movements and it is in these positions that it is so often strained.

THREE MAIN JOINTS
Actually, there are three main joints at the knee but the ordinary person just thinks of it as one; there is the chief one between the ends of the long bones of the leg, the femur and the tibia. There is also a kind of joint between the patella or kneecap and the femur. And there is the least known and thought about of them all: the point where the two bones of the calf area join: the tibiofibular joint. All these joints are subject to injury and strain and when they are not operating normally they can interfere with the mobility of the whole body.

There is a good deal of free play in the main joint of the knee when it is in a normal condition; it is able to move slightly sidewise and in rotation when the weight is taken off it and in most cases of injury and strain this free movement is lost. The parts affected may be the ligaments, the muscles, the cartilage, or a combination of them but the result is always the loss of free movement and limping movement with a straight leg.

The important thing to remember about all forms of treatment is that it has not been entirely successful unless it has restored the free movement to the joint. One can, to a certain extent, test this free movement for oneself. Stand with the affected foot about a foot in front of the other and then bend it at the knee joint. Place the hand on the top of the knee and then make a wide circle with the knee, moving it sideways as well. If the knee is properly free the easy free movement can be felt and it will be painless. When a strain has not been properly cleared up the movement of the knee will be considerably restricted.

Incidentally, this is a very good exercise for restoring the full mobility to the knee joint and should be used after any kind of strain. The danger of restricted movement in the joint lies in the fact that it may lead to arthritis. It is not an uncommon thing to hear people relate the first signs of this trouble to an accident of some kind and the knee, in particular, is likely to suffer in this way. While every effort should be made in all cases to regain the full free movement of the knee joint, where there is any tendency to rheumatism or arthritis the need to do so is imperative.

The free movement of the knee cap is very important and it may be lost through a minor injury. There is very little movement in the knee cap when the knee is bent; when the leg is straightened and the muscles relaxed there is very free movement in it which the patient can test for himself. With the fingers one can move it in several directions and this is a test of its normality. This movement must be achieved before the knee can be bent. If for any reason immediately after a strain the knee cap is fixed, no attempt must be made to forcibly bend the knee. When the leg is pressed backward in the standing position the large muscles of the thigh will strongly contract and tend to pull the knee cap upwards. This is a valuable test and exercise.

UPPER TIBIOFIBULAR

Many cases of knee troubles are not properly managed because the treatment has been directed to the main joint of the knee whereas the real difficulty lies in the upper tibiofibular joint. Many laymen, indeed, do not realize that they have such a joint but it can easily be demonstrated to them. If, in the sitting position, they cross one knee over the other and then place the thumb on the top of the uppermost knee, with the fingers reaching down the outside of the leg, they will be able to feel a slight bony lump. If now they swing the foot in various directions they will feel the joint moving under the fingers. If this joint is quite free the movement can be plainly felt but in many cases, especially where the ankle has been strained, less movement of the joint will be experienced.

The free movement of this joint may also be elicited in the following manner. In the sitting position place the heel of the foot on the floor with the front of the foot raised. Now move the foot from side to side and with the fingers feel the movement in the joint. One can test as well as exercise the joint in this way and after an ankle strain the free movement of this joint should always be ascertained.

Although one may speak of the joints and their movements in isolation, it should always be remembered that joints greatly influence each other. This is especially true of the knee. Its movements are closely associated with the movements of the hip and the ankle and this should always be taken into consideration when managing strains and minor injuries.

THE HIP JOINT

The hip joint is of the ball-and-socket variety and a pretty near perfect one of its kind. Because of its great importance in locomotion and weight-bearing any kind of disability affecting it upsets the whole balance and posture of the body. The hip joints are particularly important in relation to the erect position of the body. In this position the entire weight of the pelvis and all the parts of the body above it rests on the heads of the bones at the hip joints. When we move the body as in walking, the force and direction of the movement is initiated at the hip joint in response to the change in the head balance, with the upper part of the body to follow: all of which is dependent on the free, easy movement of the hip joints.

The hip joint plays a very important part in the posture and balance of the body. The joint is surrounded with dense fibrous tissue, which are thickened in parts to form ligaments. One of these is known as the Y-ligament because of its shape and, although few people seem aware of its function in maintaining the balance of the body, it can be shown to be of the first importance. It is attached to the pelvic bone and its purpose is to prevent excessive movement backward of the thigh on the trunk. Owing to the presence of this ligament we are able to stand in the erect position for prolonged periods without suffering from muscular fatigue.

When we stand to attention with the muscles tense and contracted we are using up a great deal of nervous energy which will lead to exhaustion; when we stand at ease we release that muscular tension and let the powerful ligament take over with the result that we can maintain that position almost indefinitely without fatigue.

OSTEOARTHRITIS

The hip joint is well protected by powerful muscles and is not liable to easy strain. It takes great violence to dislocate it, but in advanced age when the bones are brittle it is very liable to fracture. It is sometimes difficult to decide whether the fall caused the break or whether the brittle bones caused the fall. In any case, it is often the cause of a great deal of disability in later life. But the main problem with the hip joint is osteoarthritis, which because of the importance of the joint in body balance and posture and in other ways, places the sufferer under the greatest difficulties. And the fact also that it is the great weight-bearing joint of the system makes it liable to much pain and discomfort.

The question may often be asked, why does osteoarthritis settle in this joint? There are probably many factors in an industrial society which may affect the integrity of such a joint and be the first cause of its eventual breakdown. Theoretically, heavy occupations, or work in which great strain is placed on the joint, thus causing a breakdown of its cartilage, might be an important causative factor, and since it is a weight-bearing joint, body overweight might also tend to have the same effect. Of course, it may well be that the tissues of the joint have lost their resistance to disease through faulty nutrition, but it is certain that mechanical factors do sometimes enter the problem. There is also the theory that osteoarthritis may be due to an infective process which might result in the destruction of the cartilage, but nothing definite has been forthcoming in this respect.

Although it is broadly asserted that arthritis is not an inherited disease there is no doubt that it seems to run in families, which may be more a matter of similar environment rather than of inheritance. It is something which every individual should bear in mind, especially when a strain or injury has affected any joint in the body. It seems certain that where there is a family predisposition to rheumatism and arthritis the possibility of developing such a complaint in such a condition is very real. Which means that in cases of this kind the sufferer·must make doubly sure that the affected joint is fully restored to normal function.

PREVENTION THE REAL ANSWER

It is true that surgery has made great advances in the fitting of artificial hip joints but with 13 per cent of the adult population afflicted it stands to reason that the demand will soon outrun the supply. The fact is that the only real answer to this problem lies in prevention, and everything must be done to prevent undue damage to the joint, either by athletic activity, occupational stresses and strains, and whatever may be thought to have an adverse mechanical effect upon it. Above all, the free movement of the joint must be checked and maintained from time to time so that the complaint is prevented from getting a foothold which would lead to the development of the disease and all the pain, discomfort and the disability that go with it.

There is a simple test-exercise that should be used to elicit the free movement in the joint. Stand with the feet about a foot apart. Keep the one leg quite straight and then raise the foot off the floor and turn it as far as possible inwardly and then outwardly. To make the effect of the movement known to oneself, place the hand at the side of the body on the part where one can feel the hip bone and as the exercise is being done one can feel the rotation taking place. Then do the test with the other leg. When the hip joint is normal there is a full rotation of the foot; if that is limited one should find out the reason and if possible have it corrected.

To help extension of the hip or backward movement of the leg: lie on the stomach and with the leg quite straight lift it as high as possible. Relax and do the same with the other leg.

Many people feel as soon as the word arthritis is mentioned that they should adopt a fatalistic attitude about it. This is quite wrong. By attending to nutrition and by sensible exercise to keep the joints free nature will often do a good restoration job.

THE ANKLE AND FOOT
In thinking of the ankle joint and the strains and minor injuries that may affect it, one must also take into consideration the foot, since all their functions are so closely related. The foot is an arched structure and the bone of the calf, the tibia, fits on to the central bone of the arch, forming a hinge joint. The movement of the joint here is quite free in the backward and forward positions but is limited in the side to side ones. The huge weight of the body then is posed on the central bone of the arch from where it is distributed to the other twenty-five bones of the foot which are arranged in a series of arches. This gives us some twenty-four joints in the foot which makes

possible many complex movements. Of these we might say that three major ones are of the most importance to the individual, the ankle, the mid-arch and the toes.

The importance and vulnerability of the ankle joint and those of the feet is due to the fact that in addition to the bearing of the whole weight of the body, they are directly involved in the propulsion of it. When the ankle joint is strong and free and the arch of the foot flexible and springlike the posture will be well balanced and every movement will be graceful and meaningful. But strains and minor injuries may so reduce the efficiency of these structures that the very opposite may occur. The ankle joint may be limited in movement and the foot will be flattened with its springlike action completely lost. The walk may then be more of a shuffle, a condition easily identified on the streets of every city.

How does this condition of the ankle joint and the foot develop? With some young children the arch of the foot never properly develops and they go through life with a tendency to flat feet and weak ankles. But in the majority of cases the trouble develops in later life and is, generally speaking, due to strain and minor injuries of the ankles and the feet that have never been properly treated. What has happened is that the weight of the body is not carried with the foot pointing straight ahead as it should but with the front part of the foot turned outward. The result of this is that the weight then comes down on the inside of the foot and on the joint of the big toe, starting up all the foot troubles from pain and discomfort to the development of a bunion.

One can easily demonstrate this condition for oneself. Stand with the toes quite straight and see how the weight comes down, as it should, on the outside of the foot with the minimum of weight on the big toe. Now turn the feet outwards and see how the weight comes on the inside of the feet, on the spring of the arch, as it were. Then turn the feet inwards and this will throw too much weight on the outside of the foot. These movements should convince us of the fact that the best position for the feet is that of pointing directly forward.

CIRCULATION IMPEDED

If a strained ankle has wrongly adjusted its weight bearing function and partially flattened the foot, we may be sure that the effects of it will be felt in other parts of the body. It is not enough, therefore, to merely strap up a strained joint and rest it until the pain has gone; full restoration of the function of the joint means that it must regain fully its free movement and that the arch of the foot has been restored to its normal condition. If this is not done then some degree of arthritis may develop in the ankle joint and the feet. When the foot loses its elasticity, not only does it interfere with the effective movement of the whole body, but it does also impede in some way the circulation, and sufferers may often find that they are liable to be afflicted with cold feet. It is probably no exaggeration to say that the majority of adults are suffering from foot troubles of one kind or another.

To add to this, we have the problem of footwear, and all the perplexities to be met in fitting the human foot. Unfortunately, fashion and other considerations receive more attention than the anatomy of the foot. High heels strain not only the feet and the ankle joints but almost the whole of the body and may be the cause of backache. Even at best when we have fitted the most flexible and suitable of footwear, we must remember that for many hours of the day the ankles and the many joints of the feet are enclosed and under some restraint. We have all felt that sense of freedom when we remove our shoes which should remind us of the imprisonment which we constantly inflict upon them. To give the feet more freedom of movement as many young people are doing today will greatly help to decrease foot troubles in the future.

THE ELBOW JOINT

The elbow, meaning the 'bend' in the arm, is a very

complicated joint, and that is why it may give so much trouble when it has been fractured. It is very liable to strains and the so called 'tennis elbow' is, generally speaking, due to that cause. A similar condition is sometimes referred to as 'golfer's elbow' and both are probably due to strain and misuse. They can be incapacitating and annoying and sometimes resist protracted treatment. In such cases the free play movement of the joint has been lost and until that is fully restored the trouble will persist. The use of heat and suitable relaxation of the affected muscles will be found to be of great benefit in restoring the joint to its normal condition.

Symptoms similar to 'tennis elbow' and 'golfer's elbow' may arise from activities other than the playing of these games. Any twisting movement of the arm and wrist may produce strain at the elbow joint to be followed by a good deal of pain. The muscles around the joint will become tense and tender. From then onwards the patient will find it very difficult, until the normal function of the joint has been restored to its normal freedom, to use a screwdriver or to make any rotary movement of the arm that calls for muscular resistance.

It is easy to feel the movement of the elbow joint when the arm is being turned: place the fingers over the outer part of the arm at the elbow and slowly turn the hand when the motion can be plainly felt. It is this free movement that has been lost when the joint has been strained and the trouble has not been completely cleared up until it has been fully restored.

Other serious afflictions may affect the elbow joint, including, of course, arthritis, which can be both painful and incapacitating. The same rules for its avoidance apply to it as to the other joints and to preserve the full movement of the joint is undoubtedly one of the main points to keep in mind.

'MINER'S ELBOW'

There is at the elbow joint a bursa that may sometimes

swell and give rise to anxiety as to its nature. It may occur as a result of pressure on the tip of the elbow bone and resembles very much the housemaid's knee swelling that is found near the knee. Years ago it used to be known as 'miner's elbow' because of the fact that in that occupation so much resting on the joint was done. It is said that those who are liable to suffer from gout are more likely to develop this bursa swelling. It gives no real cause for alarm, and, generally speaking tends to resolve itself if treated with hot and cold applications. And, of course, the avoidance of the pressure on the joint.

THE WRIST JOINT AND HAND

The erect position of the body gave to the human two great advantages: a greater range for his sight and the possibility of developing what is perhaps the most perfect instrument, the wrist and hand — more than any other part of his body the true hallmark of mankind. The hand has developed to the point where it may perform the most delicate of manipulations; to give to man the ability to translate into concrete terms the concepts of his fertile and creative mind. Even more than that, the hand is used as a means of expression and communication: it can express thoughts and feelings almost as well as the voice, as the deaf and dumb language shows. The world of acting would be very much the poorer if it had not the practised hand to make all the gestures that the actor requires to emphasize his moods from drama to comedy.

The hand represents so many other things. The male and female hand shows plainly the differing features of both sexes, and even the character and mode of life peculiar to each individual. The hand adapts itself to the occupation of its owner; the toughened and thickened hand of the heavy worker is a clear indication of how this adaptability comes about. Each person has his own individual finger-print, and we are told that the lines on the hand may indicate the temperament and personality of the owner. Some would have us believe that they may hold the secrets of his future destiny and fortune. The artist has so often seen in the human hand its beauty which he has many times portrayed on his canvases.

It is when we see this perfect instrument deformed almost out of all recognition of its normal condition by arthritis that we realize how much damage this disease can do to this part of the body. The deformity spreads through all the joints, the muscles are wasted and around the joints there are unsightly swellings. It is plain to see how much pain and agony has been suffered before this stage of the disease has been reached. The really healthy hand has a 'personality' of its own; here we see it literally broken and ruined. Of course, the disease can and does cause deformity in other parts of the body but somehow it is in the hands, that are constantly exposed to view, that we see the disease in its destructive attack.

ARTHRITIS THE OLDEST DISEASE?

Arthritis is probably the oldest form of disease from which the human has suffered. It has been known and treated by medicine since records were kept. No one can complain that we have not had time to understand its nature and its consequences. Nor indeed has there been any lack of material for the number of people suffering from it has always been high and in practically every country. Every conceivable kind of treatment has been tried for the complaint and it would fill a large book to cover half of them. None has survived and today research is still very much at square one. At an annual meeting of the Rotal College of Physicians in 1972 a Government spokesman told the audience that 'the largest single cause of disability in this country is arthritis. There are a million severely disabled and three million mildly disabled. Arthritis is the biggest single crippler of that lot . . . '. He went on to say that research centres were operating in almost every big city and that millions of money was being spent on research. But he emphasized that 'none of this work can produce quick results'. And while he said that over ten thousand hip replacements were being done in a year and surgical techniques likely to increase, no one can pretend to think that this can be the real solution to arthritis.

In all of these crippled cases the joints of the body are the focal point for the disease and we may be quite sure that the wrist and the hand will be involved in the majority of cases. And in many ways the loss of function in the wrists and hands constitute one of the most crippling effects. So many actions that are deployed in daily tasks are essential in work and hobbies. Even in bed-ridden people who cannot use other joints of the body, the use of the hands can still give them much pleasure and indeed enable them to undertake useful jobs such as sewing and knitting.

There is no doubt that if trouble with the wrists and hands are taken in the early stages, and there are plenty of warning signs, very much can be done to prevent the loss of function in the joints. The real danger lies in making use of pain-killers like aspirin to alleviate the pain, and doing nothing fundamental to arrest the progress of the disease. It takes years to produce crippled and deformed hands and time lost in the early stages will make recovery much more difficult.

'MAN IN MINIATURE'

There are, of course, numerous joints in the wrist and hands and we should take a brief look at them to see how they work and how they can be affected. The 'hand is the man in miniature' and it is therefore worth examining very carefully for the information which it can give. The four basic functions of the hand are given as: pinch-grip, as in picking up a pin; key-grip, as in turning a key; the hammer-grip and pen-grip. How well these may be done gives one an indication of how much loss of function has taken place. On the back of the hand we can see the tendons under the skin, especially in thin and elderly people. Early signs of arthritis may be observed in this region of the hand, which may show as a swelling of the tendon sheath. Nodes develop over the tendons occasionally and, of course, the nodules are often seen near the finger joints.

In the wrist itself there are some sixteen synovial joints, but the main joints which move in it are of three kinds: flexion or forward bending, extension or backward bending and rotation-side-bending as a combined movement. In the normal wrist there is a very free movement which one can test for oneself. It can be bent backward and forward very easily and freely moving, but when the hand is rotated the movement comes from the forearm and the elbow. This gives one the extra power needed to turn a screwdriver and such other actions. A good way to test the free movement in the wrist is to grip the arm just below the wrist and hold it firmly. Now move the wrist and hand in all directions. It is surprising how free and extensive these movements can be and how important they are in giving the hand its efficiency.

The wrist is subject to many forms of strain and some of these movements may be lost if the injury is not properly treated and the full movement regained. When, as so often happens, arthritis develops following such a condition, the wrist may become partially fixed, and if the trouble is not arrested the loss of movement may become complete, with all the disadvantages to the hand movement which this entails. The stage is then set for the development of the deformed hand.

In the hand and fingers there are numerous joints, normally, all these movements are very free; it is worth testing the joints of the fingers to see how free they are when relaxed. One can bend and rotate them but when they have been strained or are arthritic they become very stiff and, in bad cases, immobile. Then the real deformity begins to show itself. The joints become buckled and the fingers are pulled to one side to such an extent in severe cases that the joints are drawn out of place. The tissues around the joints are greatly swollen and very tender. Arthritic patients are liable to suffer from what is sometimes called carpal tunnel syndrome. This means that the nerve has been suppressed, giving rise to pain, numbness and tingling, which may lead on to surgery in severe cases.

A point about the hand that is not often understood is that, like the foot, the normal hand forms an arch when it is relaxed. This can be demonstrated by placing the relaxed hand on a flat surface. It will be seen that the centre of the hand is elevated. If pressure is put on the hand the fingers and the thumb will tend to slightly separate and the palm will be forced on to the surface. When the pressure is released the centre of the hand will rise and the arch re-formed.

RIGID HAND

Rigidity of the hand can take place just as it does of the foot, and in the latter case it is recognized and called flat foot. The result is very much the same in both cases. All the joints, numerous as they are, suffer as a consequence. There will be considerably less movement in all the joints of the fingers and the thumb. In time this will mean that the flexibility of the joints will be lost and changes are certain to take place in the tissues surrounding them. Lack of movement in the wrist, a rigid palm with none of the springlike action of the arch, and stiff finger joints will surely lay the foundation for the formation of the lumpy joints and the deformity of the whole hand.

These conditions do not come on overnight. There are plenty of warning signs of the future trouble and that is the time to take the matter in hand. Experience has shown that in many cases the joints of the thumbs seem to become the seat of the arthritis in the early stages, and this will interfere, not only with the movement of the thumb, but also of many other joints. In time, and without proper treatment, the thumb joints will enlarge and lose their movement; this will prevent the stretching movement of the thumb and draw it in towards the palm. Few people past the age of fifty-five or so, still have the full

stretch-movement of the thumbs and their early implica-
tion in arthritic change is a warning of what will happen to
the rest of the hand if effective measures are not taken in
time.

When we think about the joints of the body and the
ways they are affected in health and disease, we must not
think of them in isolation. Their main function is in free
movement but they and their surrounding tissues have to
be supplied with nerve energy and with a blood supply to
bring to them their essential nutriment and to take away
the waste products of cell activity. The proper nutrition of
the body is therefore closely involved. From that standpoint suitable food and its digestion is at the base of all the
functions in the body, and with arthritis Dr Tilden, the
doyen of all nature-cure physicians, went so far as to say
that no one ever had a node on the fingers who had not
had indigestion. Unfortunately, people who do suffer from
indigestion rarely change their food to avoid it: they fly to
the usual anti-acid remedies and nothing more harmful
could be done in upsetting the alkaline-acid balance in the
body, thus directly contributing to the rheumatic and
arthritic complaints.

ALKALINE-ACID BALANCE
Disturbing the alkaline-acid balance in the body is undoubtedly a more potent cause of rheumatism and arthritis
than many people imagine and in the conventional diet
this is more often the case than otherwise. Generally
speaking, the balance is tipped over the acid side by the
use of the acid-forming foods, the proteins, meat, fish,
etc., and the free use of the refined and over-concentrated
starchy and sugary foods. The antidote to this kind of
food is to take far more generously the ripe fruits, raw
salads and cooked vegetables. These are the alkaline foods
that will help to restore the alkaline-acid balance in the
body. The best way to use these foods for their most
effective results is to make use of the fruits for breakfast,
the salads for lunch, and the cooked vegetables for the

evening meal. They should form the basis of the meals and other foods like meat, fish, eggs, cheese, should be added in small quantities. A glass of milk with the fruit meal can be taken if desired, but all the sweets, cakes, pastries, chocolate, cocoa, and all foods made with white sugar and white flour rigorously avoided. If the trouble is really severe, and more rapid results desired, the fruit, salads and cooked vegetables only should be taken for three to four days or perhaps a week. It is surprising how much grateful relief such a diet will give to the painful spasms of arthritis.

The juice of a lemon and/or a grapefruit should be taken every day, and in this respect it is well to bear in mind that the acid of such fruits are alkaline in the body. Few people seem to realize this fact and often think that the acid of fruits will produce acid within the system. It is helpful in this way to make free use of lemon juice when dressing salads, which is always preferable to the use of vinegar. Lemon juice is rich in natural vitamin C whereas vinegar, being acetic acid, is devoid of vitamins, and indeed, of any actual food value. Arthritic patients benefit from a generous amount of vegetable oil and the best way of using it is with the salads. It mixes very well with the lemon juice and adds useful nutriment to the meal. Too often mishaped and deformed hands are the outward and visible signs of mistaken habits of eating and impaired nutrition.

NATURE'S LUBRICATION
People sometimes say that they wish they could lubricate their joints, but what they forget is that nature had already provided a very efficient method of lubrication. Joints and all the other movable structures in the body are lubricated by what is known as the synovial fluid. Not only is this an efficient method of lubrication, but it is so arranged that it is most suitable for joint cavities, the tendon sheaths and the bursae wherever the need is found. This lubricating fluid is a colourless, viscid liquid consisting, among other things, of minerals and a certain kind of protein which gives it its lubricating properties.

Now this lubricating fluid has to be made in the body from the water, minerals and other foods that we take into it. It follows then that unless we do supply the body with the essential elements some deficiency will be found in the synovial fluid. And deficiency in the lubricating fluid will result in poor movements of the joints, with pain and friction. So that when this takes place the first thing that we should think about is whether the food we subsist upon is adequate to meet the demands of the system. We cannot remedy such a situation with medicines, and that is why the taking of those like aspirin, although they may ease the pain, do nothing to supply the body with its essential nutritional needs.

From this standpoint we can see how the nutritional problem can be the most important element in any form of treatment, and also see that, provided no structural change has taken place in a joint, the change to better nutrition can lead to recovery from the complaint. The importance of nutrition cannot be over-stressed. Without food we starve to death; with inadequate food we suffer from deficiency diseases; with adequate and good food we build up the health and resistance of the body and give it its best chance of recovering, not only from arthritis, but from every other form of disease.

HOT AND COLD TREATMENT

Local treatment of the joints of the wrist and hands can be of the greatest help in the treatment of strains, minor injuries and arthritis. It can assist in mobilizing and restoring joint movement; it can stimulate the circulation, helping in the circulation of the blood and other fluids and thus improving the nutrition of the tissues and cells and aid in the elimination of the waste products of cell activity. With patience and persistence much can be done to prevent the deformity of the hands from which so many people suffer at the present time.

Two essential things are required in local treatment: the application of heat and cold to the surfaces of the parts affected with the trouble and the restoration of free movements of the joints. The application of heat and cold can best be done through the use of water and in the treatment of the wrists and hands its application is, of course, very simple. There are one or two things to remember about these applications. Heat is a vital stimulant; cold is a depressant. To a certain extent we see these factors in action around us. The heat of the sun stimulates life into action; the cold season depresses it. We can use them for the same purpose on the surface of the body. Heat dilates the blood vessels and stimulates the circulation, thus assisting in the nutritive processes and the eliminative ones. Cold constricts the blood vessels and gives back tone to the tissues.

ADDED SUBSTANCES

It is the action of heat and cold on the body which is the important thing. Through their medium we get the system to act and react. And water is used for the purpose because of its simplicity and effectiveness and not because it has any special virtue. This raises the question as to whether there is any value in adding substances to the water? All manner of substances have been used, from Epsom salts to peat, mud and so on. There are two questions to be asked about them: do they improve upon hot and cold water in producing the actions and reactions of the system, and do they provide the system with some beneficial substances that is absorbed through the skin? No one has ever demonstrated that they do more than water in producing the reactions of the system – the whole purpose of the exercise. The question of absorption is still more dubious. If they do supply the system with any element of nutrition, then this could be more properly supplied to the body through the normal channels of digestion. If they act at all, one is obliged to think it is through suggestion and the inducement which they give to people of making use of heat and cold.

Experience has shown that the treatment can be made

quite effective by the use of hot and cold water — but if a person finds that the addition of a harmless substance acts as an inducement to use the water no one is likely to interfere. For the wrists and the hands the wash-basin is quite sufficient. The water should be as hot as can be reasonably borne and the hands should be immersed for about ten minutes. By that time there should be a flush on the skin showing the increase in the circulation. A basin of cold water should be nearby so that the hands may be dipped for a minute into it, which will bring the skin back to its normal colour. The hands should be thoroughly dried and a little vegetable oil well massaged into the skin. When the hands are in the hot water it is a good plan to press the hands firmly on the bottom of the wash-basin in order to spread the fingers and loosen the joints. The heat of the water softens the tissues and makes the stretching of the muscles and tendons much easier.

FINGER AND HAND EXERCISES

Many people who exercise the rest of the body often forget to exercise the hands. It is very important to do so. A useful plan is as follows: place the hands together as in prayer with the tips of the fingers and thumbs together. Now press all the tips together and then open the hands by raising the elbows. Then lower the elbows pressing the palms together. This puts pressure on all the muscles and joints of the fingers and the thumbs.

A way of testing and exercising the fingers is to grip the thumb of the left hand by the right hand. Then give the thumb a series of short tugs, sensing at the same time the movement of the joints. Do this with all the fingers of the left hand and then change over and do the right hand in the same way. If this movement is done properly, with the fingers relaxed, the free movement of the joints can be plainly felt if the joints are normal. Where there is arthritis this free movement will be lost. The main object of the testing and exercise is to restore this free movement.

Do not underestimate these simple measures. Proper

nutrition, exercise and the application of heat and cold, may be a little more troublesome than just swallowing a pill, but they are more effective and always without danger — something which one can never say about the taking of medicines.

THE JAW JOINT

This joint, to which the anatomists apply the formidable term 'temporomandibular joint', does not, as a rule, cause much trouble, but it can be the seat of pain that may be attributed to other parts of the neck and head. The joint has very free movement. It can move in three directions, opening and closing, from side to side and there is a certain degree of movement back and forward. In some people the jaw movement may make an audible clicking sound which may signify very little and is not necessarily a sign of arthritis.

It can be strained in many ways. By yawning, by biting on a hard substance, by rough usage in dental work and so on. Badly fitting dentures may impose a strain on it that is not always recognized. The pain from these strains may be easily misinterpreted. It may be passed off as a touch of rheumatism or neuralgia. Unless the strain is properly cleared up it may leave the joint limited in movement and subject to an attack of arthritis.

The joint should be tested from time to time for its free movement, which the person can easily do for himself. Placing the fingers over the face just in front of the ears and opening and shutting the mouth gives one a good idea of what the free movements should be. By cupping the hands under the jaw the movements can be resisted and the joint carefully exercised. If, as might unfortunately be the case, there are signs of arthritis developing no time should be lost in using the hot and cold applications to arrest its progress.

This joint is a good example of the way in which nature practises economy in the human system. When we use the jaw as we do in speaking, almost every moment of the day, the movement of the jaw is very limited, and therefore places very little effort on the muscles involved. When we eat and the jaws have to be moved against much more resistance, the stronger muscles take up the strain. This is a good example of the way in which nature has so carefully balanced all the functions of the system.

Summary

All the joints of the body are constantly at risk from strains and minor injuries.

Joints get better from such conditions without having the full function of the joint restored.

The test for full function of a joint is free-play movement within it. This comes from relaxation rather than from exercise.

Tests and simple movements enable the individual to judge for himself.

A joint not restored to full function is most likely to prove to be a focal point for the development of rheumatism and arthritis.

The basis of the health and resistance of the joints of the body is sound nutrition, which comes from the selection of good and adequate food.

Good food and nutrition is a vital necessity in the restoration of health and strength of joints after strains and minor injuries.

Pain and discomfort, attendant upon strains and minor injuries to joints, can best be met by natural measures rather than by the use of pain-killing drugs which should always be kept to a minimum.

A more optimistic attitude should be adopted about arthritic joints and the possibility of keeping them useful and in action by natural measures.

Joint disabilities are a major factor in causing pain and a loss of work and activity in all walks of life.